HAWAIIAN NONI

(Morinda citrifolia)

Prize Herb of Hawaii and the South Pacific

Rita Elkins, M.H.

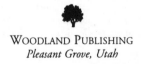

WOODLAND PUBLISHING
Pleasant Grove, Utah

CONTENTS

HAWAIIAN NONI

(Morinda citrifolia)

INTRODUCTION

I n a time when we are more concerned than ever with issues of health, noni, a tried and true tropical herb needs to be added to our list of the best natural remedies. Its usage over hundreds of years supports its description as possessing a veritable panacea of therapeutic actions. Noni's emergence as an effective natural healing agent is a timely one; herbs like noni are in high demand for their natural pharmaceutical properties in a time when cancer rates are soaring, degenerative diseases are widespread, and bacteria and viral strains are increasingly resistant to contemporary treatments. Unquestionably, all of us want to know how to:

- protect ourselves from toxins and pollutants
- prevent the premature onset of age-related diseases such as arthritis, heart disease, diabetes and stroke
- boost our immune defenses to protect from new viral and bacterial strains that have become antibiotic-resistant
- reduce our risk of developing cancer
- better digest our food for proper assimilation

Noni has the potential to boost the immune system, inhibit tumor growth, normalize physiological functions on a cellular level, and stimulate cell regeneration. Noni appears to have the ability to augment immune defenses, fight pain, reduce inflammation, and purge the intestinal system without the dangerous side effects of harsh drugs. Its impressive and widespread use among various native cultures of tropical island regions supports the theory that it possesses valuable, therapeutic compounds.

Genus

Rubiaceae

Common Names

Indian Mulberry (India), Noni (Hawaii), Nono (Tahiti and Raratonga), Polynesian Bush Fruit, Painkiller Tree (Caribbean islands), Lada (Guam), Mengkudo (Malaysia), Nhau (Southeast Asia), Grand Morinda (Vietnam), Cheesefruit (Australia), Kura (Fiji), Bumbo (Africa)

This is only a small sampling of vernacular names for Morinda citrifolia. Almost every island nation of the South Pacific and Caribbean has a term for this particular plant. This booklet will refer to the herb mainly as "noni" or "*M. citrifolia,*" and is referring primarily to Hawaiian noni.

Parts Used

Every part of the noni plant is useful: the seeds have a purgative action, the leaves are used to treat external inflammations and relieve pain, the bark has strong astringent properties and can treat malaria, the root extracts lower blood pressure, the flower essences relieve eye inflammations—but the fruit, with its numerous pharmaceutical actions, is the most valuable portion of the noni plant.

Physical Description

Morinda citrifolia is technically an evergreen shrub or bush, which can grow to heights of fifteen to twenty feet. It has rigid, coarse branches which bear dark, oval, glossy leaves. Small white fragrant flowers bloom out of cluster-like pods which bear creamy-white colored fruit. The fruit is fleshy and gel-like when ripened, resembling a small breadfruit. The flesh of the fruit is characteristically bitter, and when completely ripe produces a rancid and very distinctive odor. Noni has buoyant seeds that can float for months in water. The wood of the *Morinda* tree is known for its hardness, resistance to salt and very lovely grain.

Character

Noni can be considered an antibacterial, analgesic, anticongestive, antioxidant, anticatarrhal, anti-inflammatory, astringent, emollient, emmenagogue, laxative, sedative, hypotensive (lowers blood pressure), blood purifier, and tonic.

Chemical Constituents

Noni has various chemical constituents. First, it has an impressive array of terpene compounds, three of which—*L. Asperuloside*, aucubin, and glucose—have been identified by their acetyl derivatives. Both caproic and caprylic acids have been isolated.[1] Second, bushfruits, a category of which noni fruit is a member, are also considered a good source of vitamin C.[2] Third, Hawaiian noni has been linked to the synthesis of xeronine in the body which has significant and widespread health implications. Last, the alkaloid content of the noni fruit is thought to be responsible for its therapeutic actions. Alkaloids exhibit a wide range of pharmacological and biological activities in the human body. They are nitrogen-containing organic compounds that react with acids to form salts, which are the basis of many medicines. Finally, the ezymatic actions of noni make it valuable as a health promoter in cells. The following is an in-depth chemical analysis of each plant part and its chemical constituents:

LEAF

- amino acids (which include alanine, arginine, aspartic acids, cysteine, cystine, glycine, glutamic acid, histidine, leucine, isoleucine, methionine, phenylalanine, proline, serine, threonine, tryptophan tyrosine, and valine)
- anthraquinones
- glycosides
- phenolic compounds
- resins
- B-sitosterol
- ursolic acid

FLOWER

- acacetin 7-0-D (+)-glucophyranoside
- 5,7,-dimethyl apigenin-4-0-8-D(+)-galactophyranoside
- 6,8,-dimethoxy-3-methyl anthroquinone-1-0-8-rhamnosyl glucophyranoside

FRUIT

- antioxidant
- alizarin

- anthraquinones
- caproic and caprylic acids
- essential oil
- B-D-glucopyranose pentaacetate [2]
- asperuloside tetra acetate
- glucose
- ascorbic acid (The high ascorbic acid [vitamin C] content of this bushfruit makes it a valuable food source.)[3]

Dr. Ralph Heinicke of the University of Hawaii discovered an alkaloid in the Hawaiian noni fruit which he calls *proxeronine*. Heinicke believes proxeronine has appreciable physiological benefits by acting as a precursor to xeronine, a very crucial compound (see later sections). In addition, a compound found in the fruit called damnacanthol is believed to help inhibit certain viruses and cellular mutations involved in cancer.

ROOT AND ROOT BARK

- carbonate
- rubicholric acid
- chrysophanol
- magnesium
- sodium
- morinadadiol
- resins
- sterols[4]

- chlorubin
- soranjidol
- phosphate
- ferric iron
- glycosides
- morindine
- rubiadin

Pharmacology

Recent surveys have suggested that noni fruit exerts antibiotic action. In fact, a variety of compounds which have antibacterial properties (such as aucubin) have been identified in the fruit.[5] The 6-D-glucopyranose pentaacetate of the fruit extract is not considered bacteriostatic.[6] Constituents found in the fruit portion have exhibited antimicrobial action against *Escherichia coli*, *Salmonella typhi* (and other types), *Shigella paradysenteriae*, and *Staphylococcus aureus*. Compounds found in the root have the ability to reduce swollen mucous membrane and lower blood pressure in animal studies.

Proxeronine is an alkaloid constituent found in Hawaiian noni fruit that prompts the production of xeronine in the body. Dr. Heinicke, who discovered proxeronine, theorized that this proenzyme can be effective in initiating a series of beneficial cellular reactions through its involvement with the integrity of specific proteins. He points out that tissues contain cells which possess certain receptor sites for xeronine. Because the reactions that can occur are so varied, different therapeutic actions can result when xeronine production escalates, explaining why Hawaiian noni is good for many seemingly unrelated disorders.

Damnacanthol is another compound contained in the fruit of the Hawaiian noni plant which has shown the ability to block or inhibit the cellular function of RAS cells, widely considered to be pre-cancerous cells.

Body Systems Targeted

The following body systems have all been effectively influenced by noni: circulatory, digestive, respiratory, integumentary (skin), endocrine, immune, nervous, and skeletal.

Current Forms Available

The forms of noni currently available include juice, freeze-dried capsules, dehydrated powder or fruit, and oil. Noni plant constituents are sometimes offered in combination with other herbs. Some products contain a percentage of the fruit, bark, root, and seeds for their individual therapeutic properties.

Safety

Extracts of *M. citrifolia* are considered safe if used as directed; however, pregnant or nursing mothers should consult their physicians before taking any supplement. High doses of root extracts may cause constipation. Taking noni supplements with coffee, alcohol, or nicotine is not recommended.

Suggested Uses

Ideally, noni extracts should be taken on an empty stomach prior to meals. The process of digesting food can interfere with the medicinal value of the alkaloid compounds found in Hawaiian noni, especially in its fruit. Apparently, stomach acids and enzymes destroy the specific enzyme that frees up the xeronine compound. Using supplements that have been made from the semi-ripe or light-green fruit is also considered preferable to the ripe, whitish fruit.

NONI: ITS USE AND HISTORY

Noni is a tropical wandering plant indigenous to areas of Australia, Malaysia, and Polynesia. It is considered native to Southeast Asia although it grows from India to the eastern region of Polynesia. *Morinda citrifolia* has a long history of medicinal use throughout these areas. It is thought to be the "most widely and commonly used medicinal plant prior to the European era."[7]

Centuries ago, the bushfruit was introduced to native Hawaiians, who subsequently called it "noni" and considered its fruit and root as prized medicinal agents. Among all Polynesian botanical agents of the 19th and 20th centuries, Hawaiian noni has the widest array of medical applications. Samoan and Hawaiian medical practitioners used noni for bowel disorders (especially infant diarrhea, constipation, or intestinal parasites), indigestion, skin inflammation, infection, mouth sores, fever, contusions, and sprains. Hawaiians commonly prepared noni tonics designed to treat diabetes, stings, burns, and fish poisoning.[8] The herb's remarkable ability to purge the intestinal tract and promote colon health was well known among older Hawaiian and Tahitian natives and folk healers.

Interestingly, field observations regarding noni's reputation discovered that its medical uses were frequently passed down from mother to child. Noni is intrinsically linked to the rich healing heritage of the Polynesian culture. The fact that cultures in Samoa, Tonga, the Philippines, Tahiti, India, and Guam had become familiar with *M. citrifolia* and its medical applications strongly attests to its credibility as a remarkable healing agent.

Wonder Herb of Island Folk Healers

Common to the thickets and forests of Malaysia and Polynesia, and the low hilly regions of the Philippine islands, noni has been cultivated throughout communities in the South Pacific for hundreds of years. Its Hawaiian use is thought to originate from inter-island canoe travel and settlement dating to the centuries before the birth of Christ. Its hardy seeds have the ability to float which has also contributed to its distribution among various seacoasts in the South Pacific region.

Historical investigation has established the fact that some of Hawaii's earliest settlers probably came via Tahiti. For this reason, Tahitian herbal practices have specific bearing on the herbal therapeutics of islands to the north. The very obvious similarities between the Hawaiian vernacular for herbal plants and Tahitian names strongly suggests the theory of Polynesian migrations to Hawaii.

Cultures native to these regions favored using *Morinda citrifolia* for treating major diseases and utilized it as a source of nourishment in times of famine.[9] Noni fruit has been recognized for centuries as an excellent source of nutrition. The peoples of Fiji, Samoa and Raratonga use the fruit in both its raw and cooked forms.[10] Traditionally, the fruit was picked before it was fully ripe and placed in the sunlight. After being allowed to ripen, it was typically mashed and its juice extracted through a cloth. Noni leaves provided a vegetable dish and their resiliency made them desirable as a fish wrap for cooking.

Noni's Medical Reputation

Elaborate traditional rituals and praying rites usually accompanied the administration of noni. Interestingly, cultures indigenous to the Polynesian islands had a significant understanding of their flora. For example, native Hawaiians maintained a folk-medicine taxonomy that was considered second to none.[11]

Research indicates that noni was among the few herbal remedies that islanders considered "tried and true." In Hawaii, trained herbal practitioners reserved the right to prescribe plant therapies.[12] Records indicate that Hawaiian medical practices were based on extensive and very meticulous descriptions of symptoms and their prescribed herbal treatments. Dosages were controlled and the collection and administration of plant extracts was carefully monitored.[13]

In addition to *M. citrifolia*, it was not uncommon for these herbal doctors to also recommend using papaya and kava kava, two herbs which are commonly used today.[14] Moreover, these Hawaiian medicine men also knew when and how to combine various herbal agents to achieve desired results. It was also common practice to mix plant extracts with coconut oil for external applications.

In regard to its application for common ailments, Hawaiians and other island communities traditionally prescribed noni to purge the bowel, reduce fever, cure respiratory infections such as asthma, ease skin inflammations, and heal bruises and sprains. In other words, noni was widely used and highly regarded as a botanical medicine.

A Timely Reemergence

Today, the natural pharmaceutical actions of the chemical constituents contained in noni are scientifically emerging as valuable botanical medicines. Tahitian "nono" intrigued medical practitioners decades ago. However, due to the eventual emergence of synthetic drugs, interest in this island botanical diminished until recent years. Ethnobotanists are once again rediscovering why Hawaiian people have treasured and cultivated *Morinda citrifolia* for generations. Noni is now finding its way into Western therapeutics and is referred to as "the queen" of the genus Rubiaceae. Its ability to reduce joint inflammation and target the immune system have made it the focus of the modern scientific inquiry.

Studies investigating noni as an anticancer agent have been encouraging. Its conspicuous attributes and varied uses have elevated its status to one of the best of the healing herbs. Today *Morinda citrifolia* is available in liquid, juice, freeze-dried capsules, or oil forms, and is considered one of nature's most precious botanicals.

TRADITIONAL USES OF NONI

Throughout tropical regions, virtually every part of *Morinda citrifolia* was used to treat disease or injury. Its curative properties were well known and commonly employed. Patoa Tama Benioni, a member of the Maori tribe from the Cook Islands and a lecturer on island plants, explains:

> Traditionally Polynesians use noni for basically everything in the treatment of illness. Noni is a part of our lives. Any Polynesian boy will tell you he's had experience with it. We use juice from its roots, its flowers, and its fruit . . . my grandmother taught me to use noni from the roots and the leaves to make medicine for external as well as internal use, and for all kinds of ailments, such as coughs, boils, diseases of the skin, and cuts.[15]

The following is only a partial list of how island folk healers used this very valuable plant.

- Poultices of noni fruit were applied to swollen areas, deep cuts, boils, and inflamed joints for immediate relief.
- Women in Malaysia used noni fruit juice and bark decoctions to stimulate delayed menstruation.
- Noni was frequently utilized for its antiparasitic activity.
- Respiratory ailments, coughs, and colds were treated with noni.
- A juice made from pounding noni leaves, roots and fruit mixed with water was administered for diarrhea.
- Dried and powdered forms of the bark mixed with water and administered with a spoon treated infant diarrhea.
- Small pieces of fruit and root infused with water were given to kill intestinal parasites.

- Boiled bark decoctions were given as a drink for stomach ailments.
- Coughs were treated with grated bark.
- Charred unripe fruit was used with salt on diseased gums. .
- Pounded fruit combined with kava and sugar cane was used to treat tuberculosis.
- Babies were rubbed with fresh, crushed leaves for serious chest colds accompanied by fever.
- Eye washes were made from decoctions for eye complaints from flower extracts.
- Leaf infusions were traditionally taken to treat adult fevers.
- A mouthwash consisting of crushed ripe fruit and juice was used for inflamed gums in young boys.
- Pounded leaf juice was used for adult gingivitis.
- Sore throats were treated by chewing the leaves and swallowing the juice.
- Skin abscesses and boils were covered with leaf poultices.
- Swelling was controlled with leaf macerations.
- Heated leaves were used for arthritic joins and for ringworm.[16]

XERONINE: THE SECRET OF NONI?

One informed professional on the subject of noni is Dr. Heinicke, a biochemist who has researched the active compounds of noni fruit for a number of years. He discovered that the Hawaiian noni fruit contains an alkaloid precursor to a very vital compound called xeronine. Without xeronine, life would cease.

In Dr. Heinicke's view, noni fruit provides a safe and effective way to increase xeronine levels in the body, profoundly affecting cell health and protection. His research suggests that the juice from the *M. citrifolia* fruit contains proxeronine, a precursor of the crucial compound xeronine. Proxeronine initiates the release of xeronine in the intestinal tract after it comes in contact with a specific enzyme which is also contained in the fruit. This particular chemical combination is believed to significantly affect cellular function for the positive.

Protein Regulator

Dr. Heinicke's research is based on the premise that one of the primary functions of xeronine is to regulate the shape and integrity of specific proteins. Because proteins and enzymes have so many varied roles within cell processes, the normalization of these proteins with noni supplementation could initiate a very wide variety of body responses and treat many disease conditions. Proteins are the most important catalysts found in the body. The beauty of obtaining a precursor to xeronine from the noni fruit is that the body naturally decides how much of this precursor to convert to xeronine. Disease, stress, anger, trauma and injury can lower xeronine levels in the body, thus creating a xeronine deficit. Supplementing the body with noni fruit is considered an excellent way to safely and naturally raise xeronine levels. It is the research and theories of Dr. Heinicke which have made the juice of the Hawaiian noni fruit a viable medicinal substance. He writes:

> Xeronine is an alkaloid, a substance the body produces in order to activate enzymes so they can function properly. It also energizes and regulates the body. This particular alkaloid has never been found because the body makes it, immediately uses it, and then breaks it down. At no time is there an appreciable, isolable amount in the blood. But xeronine is so basic to the functioning of proteins, we would die without it. Its absence can cause many kinds of illness.[17]

Because so many diseases result from an enzyme malfunction, Dr. Heinicke believes that using the noni fruit can result in an impressive array of curative applications. Interestingly, he believes that we manufacture proxeronine while we are sleeping. He proposes that if we could constantly supply our bodies with proxeronine from other sources, our need to sleep would diminish.[18]

NONI PROCESSING

How an herb is processed is crucial to how beneficial it is. This is especially true of noni, with its unique enzymes and alkaloids. Morinda citrifolia should be picked when the fruit is turning from its dark green immature color to its lighter green color, and certainly before it ripens to its white, almost translucent color. Once picked, noni, like aloe, will denature extremely quickly due to its very active enzymes. After harvesting, it should swiftly be flash frozen. This is similar to what is done to fish caught at sea to keep them fresh. This stops it from losing its potency while not damaging any of its constituents.

The best supplementation of noni is a freeze-dried, powdered form. The freeze-drying process removes only the water without damaging any of this plant's vital enzymes and other phytonutrients like xeronine and proxeronine. This pure high-quality noni fruit juice powder is a ten to one extract or concentrate using ten pounds of whole noni fruit to produce one pound of freeze-dried powder. This powder is then encapsulated (it is fruit juice without water!) This is important because typical noni fruit juices are 88 percent or more water; therefore you must literally drink gallons of juice to get the same benefits as the freeze-dried form. Most noni juices available on the market are commercially processed and have water, fruit juices and preservatives added to them. Traditionally noni juice has a very harsh taste and an extremely foul smell, similar to the fruit itself.

Other methods of processing include thermal processing, dehydration and air drying. Thermal processing is generally found in liquids, while the dehydrated noni is then milled and encapsulated. Unfortunately both methods utilize high heat (110° F+), which can deactivate many of the vital compounds that make noni so important. Air-drying is effective without using damaging heat but has quality control problems for commercial production.

MODERN APPLICATIONS OF NONI

Overview

Noni possesses a wide variety of medicinal properties which originate from its differing plant components. The fruit and leaves of the shrub exert antibacterial activities. Its roots promote the expulsion of mucus and the shrinkage of swollen membranes making it an ideal therapeutic for nasal congestion, lung infections, and hemorrhoids. Noni root compounds have also shown natural sedative properties as well as the ability to lower blood pressure. Leaf extracts are able to inhibit excessive blood flow or to inhibit the formation of blood clots. Noni is particularly useful for its ability to treat painful joint conditions and to resolve skin inflammations. Many people take noni fruit extracts for hypertension, painful menstruation, arthritis, gastric ulcers, diabetes, and depression. Recent studies suggest that its anticancer activity should also be considered.

Concerning the therapeutic potential of the Hawaiian noni fruit, Dr. Heinicke writes:

I have seen the compound found in noni work wonders. When I was still investigating its possibilities, I had a friend who was a medical research scientist administer the proxeronine to a woman who had been comatose for three months. Two hours after receiving the compound, she sat up in bed and asked where she was. . . . Noni is probably the best source of proxeronine that we have today.[19]

Studies and surveys combine to support the ability of noni to act as an immunostimulant, inhibit the growth of certain tumors, enhance and normalize cellular function and boost tissue regeneration. It is considered a powerful blood purifier and contributor to overall homeostasis.

Noni Juice: Molecular Miracle?

Dr. Heinicke also believes that the compounds specific to noni fruit juice work to actually repair damaged cells on a molecular level. The proxeronine content of noni boosts the body's production of xeronine, which appears to be able to regulate the shape and integrity of certain proteins that individually contribute to specific cellular activities.

Some practitioners believe that xeronine is best obtained from a noni fruit juice precursor compound. The enzymatic reactions that occur with taking the juice on an empty stomach are what Dr. Heinicke believes set cellular repair into motion.

Cancer

A study conducted in 1994 cited the anticancer activity of *Morinda citrifolia* against lung cancer. A team of scientists from the University of Hawaii used live laboratory mice to test the medicinal properties of the fruit against Lewis lung carcinomas which were artificially transferred to lung tissue. The mice that were left untreated died in nine to twelve days. However, giving noni juice in consistent daily doses significantly prolonged their life span. Almost half of these mice lived for more than fifty days.[20] Research conclusions stated that the chemical constituents of the juice acted indirectly by enhancing the ability of the immune system to deal with the invading malignancy by boosting macrophage or lymphocyte activity. Further evaluation theorized that the unique chemical constituents of *Morinda citrifolia* initiated enhanced T-cell activity, a reaction that may explain noni's ability to treat a variety of infectious diseases.[21]

In Japan, similar studies on noni extracts found that damnacanthol, a compound found in *Morinda citrifolia,* is able to inhibit the function of K-RAS-NRK cells, which are considered precursors to certain types of malignancies.[22] The experiment involved adding noni plant extract to RAS cells and incubating them for a number of days. Observation disclosed that noni was able to significantly inhibit RAS cellular function. Among 500 plant extracts, *Morinda citrifolia* was determined to contain the most effective compounds to combat RAS cells. Its damnacanthol content was clinically described in 1993 as "a new inhibitor of RAS function."[23]

The xeronine factor is also involved in that xeronine helps to normalize the way malignant cells behave. While they are still technically cancer cells, they no longer function as cells with unchecked growth. In time, the body's immune system may be able to eradicate these cells.

Arthritis

According to Dr. Heinicke's theories, the xeronine link found in Hawaiian noni fruit has the ability to "help cure various manifestations of diseases such as cancer, senility, arthritis, high blood pressure and low blood pressure."[24] Anecdotal surveys have found that noni repeatedly eases the joint pain associated with arthritic disease. One link to arthritic pain may be the inability to properly or completely digest proteins which can then form crystal-like deposits in the joints. The ability of Hawaiian noni fruit to enhance protein digestion through enhanced enzymatic function may help to eliminate this particular phenomenon.

In addition, the alkaloid compounds and plant metabolites of noni may be linked to its apparent anti-inflammatory action. Plant sterols can assist in inhibiting the inflammatory response which causes swelling and pain. In addition, the antioxidant effect of noni may help to decrease free radical damage in joint cells, which can exacerbate discomfort and degeneration.

Immune System

The alkaloid and other chemical compounds found in noni have proven themselves to effectively control or kill over six types of infectious bacterial strains, including *Escherichia coli, salmonella typhi* (and other types), *shigella paradysenteriae,* and *staphylococcus aureus.*[25] In addition, damnacanthol was able to inhibit the early antigen stage of the Epstein-Barr virus.

The bioactive components of the whole plant, combined or in separate portions, have demonstrated the ability to inhibit several different strains of bacteria. Anecdotal reports support this action in that noni seems particularly effective in shortening the duration of certain types of infection. This may explain why noni is commonly used to treat colds and flu.

The chemical constituents found in noni and the possibility that they stimulate xeronine production—as well as initiate alkaloid therapy—may explain noni's reputation for having immuno-stimulatory properties. Alkaloids have been able to boost phagocytosis which is the process in which certain white blood cells called macrophages attack and literally digest infectious organisms. Interestingly, the antitumor action of noni has been ascribed to an immune system response which involves stimulating T-cells.

Nutritive Booster

More and more research suggests that because *M. citrifolia* compounds enable the immune system to function more effectively, taking the herb in concentrated forms may significantly boost health and performance. These compounds appear to have the ability to increase the absorption, assimilation and utilization of vitamins and minerals. The presence of proxeronine in noni initiates a rise of xeronine in the intestinal tract which enables the walls of the intestines to more efficiently absorb various nutrients, especially amino acids. Vitamins act synergistically with xeronine to nourish all body systems.

In addition, leaf extracts of the plant have a significant amount of protein and the fruit contains a substantial ascorbic acid content. *M. citrifolia* fruit has been considered a food staple in Polynesia for centuries. Apparently, even soldiers stationed in tropical regions during World War II learned of the fruit's ability to boost endurance and stamina. Native cultures in Samoa, Tahiti, Raratonga, and Australia used the fruit in cooked and raw forms. *M. citrifolia* is considered a tonic and is especially recommended for debilitated conditions.

Antioxidant

The process of aging bombards the body with free radicals which can cause all kinds of degenerative diseases. The xeronine theory promoted by Dr. Heinicke submits that as our bodies age, we lose our ability to synthesize xeronine. To make matters worse, the presence of many environmental toxins actually blocks the production of xeronine. Heinicke believes that the proxeronine content of Hawaiian noni fruit juice can help to block these actions, working as an antiaging compound.[26]

The phytonutrients found in noni assist in promoting cell nourishment and protection from free radicals created by exposure to pollution and other potentially damaging agents. In addition, *Morinda citrifolia* contains selenium, one of the best antioxidant compounds available.

Diabetes

While scientific studies are lacking in this particular application of noni, Hawaiians used various parts of the plant and its fruit to treat blood sugar disorders. Anecdotal surveys have found that noni is currently recommended for anyone with diabetes.

Pain Killer

A 1990 study found that extracts derived from the *Morinda citrifolia* root have the ability to kill pain in animal experiments.[27] Interestingly, it was during this study that the natural sedative action of the root was also noted. This study involved a French team of scientists who noted a significant central analgesic activity in laboratory mice.[28] Dr. Heinicke has stated, "Xeronine also acts as a pain reliever. A man with very advanced intestinal cancer was given three months to live. He began taking the proxeronine and lived for a whole year, pain-free."[29]

Skin Healing Agent

One of the most prevalent historical uses of noni was in poultice form for cuts, wounds, abrasions, burns and bruises. Using its fruit extract for very serious burns has resulted in some extra-ordinary healing. Because skin is comprised of protein, it immediately responds to the presence of xeronine. When the skin is broken or traumatized, proxeronine enters the affected region from surrounding areas, and xeronine synthesis subsequently rises, enhancing healing and tissue regeneration. Burns are especially vulnerable to this biochemical process. Consequently, boosting xeronine production within a burn site through the direct application of a noni poultice is considered quite effective by Dr. Heinicke and his colleagues, who have studied enzymatic therapy. Concerning burns, he has written:

> I believe that each tissue has cells which contain proteins which have receptor sites for the absorption of xeronine. Certain of these proteins are the inert forms of enzymes which require absorbed xeronine to become active. This xeronine, by converting the body's procollangenase system into a specific protease, quickly and safely removes the dead tissue from burns.[30]

Drug Addiction

The xeronine link to treating drug addiction is based on the notion that flooding the brain with extra xeronine can reverse the neurochemical basis for addiction. This natural alkaloid is thought to normalize brain receptors which subsequently results in the cessation of physiological dependence on a certain chemical like nicotine.[31] The potential of Hawaiian noni as a natural stimulator for the production of xeronine may have profound implications in treating various types of addictions.

Complementary Agents of Noni

- cat's claw
- kava kava
- papaya
- pau d'arco

- bioflavonoids
- germanium
echinacea
- aloe vera
- shark cartilage

- selenium
- grapeseed extract
- proteolytic enzymes
- glucosamine

Primary Applications of Noni

- abrasions
- atherosclerosis
- boils
- burns
- chronic fatigue syndrome
- cold sores
- congestion
- depression
- eye inflammations
- fractures
- gingivitis
- high blood pressure
- indigestion
- kidney disease
- menstrual irregularities
- respiratory disorders
- sinusitis
- sprains
- tumors

- arthritis
- bladder infections
- bowel disorders
- cancer
- circulatory weakness
- colds
- constipation
- diabetes
- fever
- gastric ulcers
- headaches
- immune weakness
- intestinal parasites
- menstrual cramps
- mouth sores
- ringworm
- skin inflammation
- thrush
- wounds

CONCLUSION

There is no question that the very extensive geographical dispersal and widespread use of *Morinda citrifolia* in tropical regions attests to its credibility as a valuable herbal medicine. While more scientific study on its biochemical attributes is warranted, what has already emerged provides substantial validation of its medicinal worth. The enzymatic theories of Dr. Heinicke do warrant further study, but his research and experience have already elevated the status of the Hawaiian noni plant to that of a remarkable healing resource. What the peoples of the South Pacific have known and practiced for generations should be incorporated into our modern-day search for disease eradication, and health promotion.

ENDNOTES

1 Oscar Levand and Harold O. Larson, "Some Chemical Constituents of Morinda Citrifolia," DEPARTMENT OF CHEMISTRY, UNIVERSITIES OF GUAM AND HAWAII.

2 N. Peerzoda, S. Renaud and P. Ryan, "Vitamin C and Elemental Composition of Some Bushfruits," JOURNAL OF PLANT NUTRITION, 13 (7), 1990, 787.

3 Ibid.

4 Alexander Dittmar, "Morinda citrifolia L. Use in Indigenous Samoan Medicine," JOURNAL OF HERBS, SPICES AND MEDICINAL PLANTS, vol. 1(3), 1993, 89-91.

5 Levand.

6 Dittmar, 87.

7 Dr. Arthur W. Whistler, POLYNESIAN HERBAL MEDICINE, National Botanical Garden, Hong Kong: 1992, 174.

8 Ibid.

9 Julia F. Morton, "The Ocean-Going Noni or Indian Mulberry (Morinda Citrifolia, Rubiaceae) and Some of Its Colorful Relatives," ECONOMIC BOTANY, 46 (3), 1992, 243. See also O. Degener, PLANTS OF THE HAWAII NATIONAL PARK, New York Botanical Garden, Bronx park, NY, 1945.

10 Ibid., See also F.B.H. Brown, :Flora of southeastern Polynesia," III DICOTYLEDONS BULL., 130, Bernice P. Bishop Mus., Honolulu, Hi.

11 Isabella A. Abbot and Colleen Shimazu, "The Geographic Origin of the plants Most Commonly Used for Medicine by Hawaiians," JOURNAL OF ETHNOPHARMACOLOGY, 14, 1985, 214.

12 Ibid., 221.

13 Ibid.

14 Ibid.

15 "Dr. Heinicke and the Secrets of Noni," HEALTH NEWS, Triple R. Publishing, vol. 3, no.2, 4

16 Ibid.

17 Ibid., 2

18 Morton, 247-48.

19 HEALTH NEWS, 4.

20 A. Hirazumi, E. Furusawa, S.C. Chou and Y. Hokama, "Anticancer activity of Morinda Citrifolia on intraperiotneally implanted Lewis lung carcinoma in syngenic mice," PROC. WEST. PHARMACOL., (37), 1994, 145-46.

21 Ibid.

22 T. Hiramatsu, M. Imoto, T. Koyano and K. Umezawa, "Induction of normal phenotypes in RAS-transformed cells by damnacanthal from Morinda citrifolia," CANCER LETTERS, (73), 1993, 161-66.

23 Ibid.

24 HEALTH NEWS, 4.

25 Dittmar, 88.

26 HEALTH NEWS, 4.

27 C. Younos, A. Rolland, J. Fleurentin, et al., "Analgesic and behavioral effects of Morinda Citrifolia," PLANTA MEDICA, (56), 1990, 430-34.

28 Ibid.

29 HEALTH NEWS, 4.

30 R.M. Heinicke, "The Pharmacologically Active Ingredient of Noni," University of Hawaii and R.M/ Heinicke, "Cell Regeneration: Unlocking the Secrets of Tahitian Noni," audio tape, 1996.

31 Ibid.

Additional Sources

Baldwin, R.E., HAWAII'S POISONOUS PLANTS, The Petroglyph Press, Hilo, Hawaii, 1979.

Bryan, E.H., SAMOAN AND SCIENTIFIC NAMES OF PLANTS FOUND IN SAMOA, complied for the Governor of Samoa, Hamilton Library, University of Hawaii, 1935.

Bushnell, O.A. et al., "Antibacterial properties of some plants in Hawaii," PACIFIC SCIENCE, (4), 1950.

Burkill, I.H., DICTIONARY OF THE ECONOMIC PRODUCTS OF THE MALAY PENINSULA, Crown Agents for the Colonies, London, 1935.

Chang, P. And K.H. Lee, "Antitumor agents 75. Synthesis of cytotoxic anthraquinones digifer-rubiginol and mornindaparvin-B," JOURNAL NAT. PROD., 48 (6), 1985.

Krauss, B.H., NATIVE PLANTS USED AS MEDICINE IN HAWAII, Honolulu, 1979.

Negata, K.M. "Hawaiian Medicinal Plants," ECONOMIC BOTANY, (25), 1971.

Weiner, M. "Ethnomedicine in Tonga," ECONOMIC BOTANY, (25), 1971.

Perry, L.M., MEDICINAL PLANTS OF EAST AND SOUTHEAST ASIA: ATTRIBUTED PROPERTIES AND USES, The MIT Press, Cambridge Ma., 1980.

Merrill, Elmer Drew, POLYNESIAN BOTANICAL BIBLIOGRAPHY, 1773-1935, Bernice P. Bishop Museum, Honolulu, 1937.